Health Benefits of Cinnamon

By M. Usman

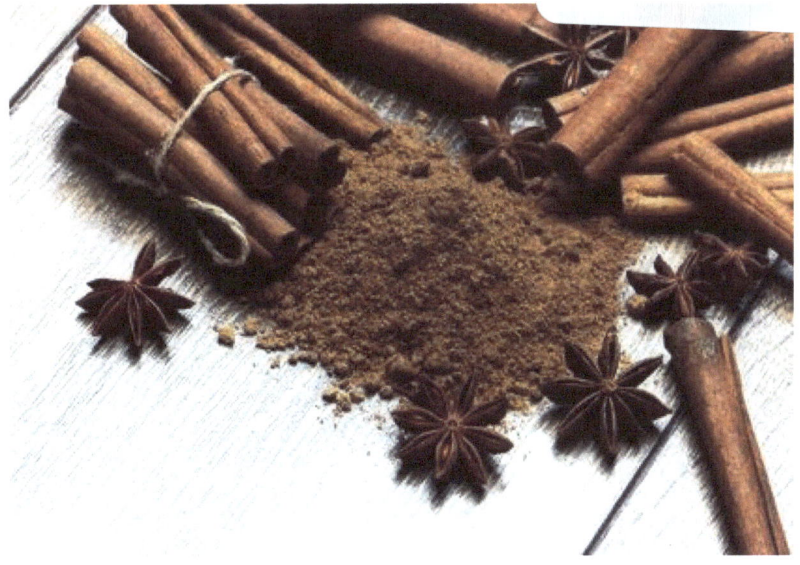

Health Learning Series

Mendon Cottage Books

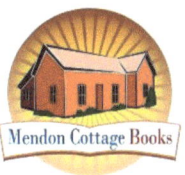

JD-Biz Publishing

Disclaimer

The information is this book is provided for informational purposes only. It is not intended to be used and medical advice or a substitute for proper medical treatment by a qualified health care provider. The information is believed to be accurate as presented based on research by the author.

The contents have not been evaluated by the U.S. Food and Drug Administration or any other Government or Health Organization and the contents in this book are not to be used to treat cure or prevent disease or mental illness.

The author or publisher is not responsible for the use or safety of any diet, procedure or treatment mentioned in this book. The author or publisher is not responsible for errors or omissions that may exist.

Warning

The Book is for informational purposes only and before taking on any diet, treatment or medical procedure it is recommended to consult with your primary care provider.

Our books are available at

1. Amazon.com
2. Barnes and Noble
3. Itunes
4. Kobo
5. Smashwords
6. Google Play Books

Table of Contents

Table of Contents...3

Preface 5

Getting Started...7

Chapter # 1: Intro...7

Chapter # 2: How is cinnamon commonly used?.....................9

Chapter # 3: Types of cinnamon 11

□ Cinnamomum verum: 11

□ Cassia cinnamon: 12

Chapter # 4: Making the most of cinnamon in daily life 14

1. Buy fresh, keep fresh: 14

2. Buy organically grown cinnamon:.......................14

3. Consume cinnamon sparingly in foods:..............15

4. Combine cinnamon in a warm drink:...................15

5. Cinnamon after meals: 16

6. Cinnamon can help when you're on a diet:..........16

7. Chew cinnamon flavored gum: 16

8. Use cinnamon in soups and drinks instead of baked goods: 17

9. Cinnamon is an anticoagulant:.............................17

10. Intake cinnamon through the air you breathe: 17

Chapter # 5: Maximum daily dosage...................................18

Benefits of cinnamon to the brain 19

Chapter # 6: Boosts brain activity................................19

Chapter # 7: Protects against Alzheimer's disease.................21

Benefits of cinnamon to the body 24

Chapter # 8: Regulates blood sugar..............................24

Chapter # 9: Aids in weight loss................................26

Chapter # 10: Helps fight cancer................................28

Chapter # 11: Combats infertility 31

Chapter # 12: Reduces arthritic pain 33

Chapter # 13: Has inherent anti-infectious properties...........35

Chapter # 14: Helps against acne................................38

Conclusion 40

Photo credits...42

Author Bio..43

Publisher...54

Preface

There is hardly anyone who does not consume spices regularly in one form or another. Spices find diverse uses ranging from natural flavor enhancement and brain simulation to traditional herbal medicine. There was a time when the spice trade was considered the most profitable and lucrative business by merchants who sailed from the West to the Indies.

There is a plethora of extremely beneficent spices out there but the one particular spice this book is concerned with is cinnamon. Procured from the internal bark of many trees belonging to the genus Cinnamomum, it is has an international reputation as an integral part of many sweet and savory foods.

What most people don't realize is that this miraculous spice is truly a gift of nature. It has amazing benefits that go far beyond its pleasant taste and aroma. Recent studies in universities and medical research centers from around the world have proven what traditional herbalists claimed for ages: Cinnamon has powerful medicinal applications that are diverse as they are many. Its positive effects on the human physiology include those on both the mind and the body.

This book contains information regarding cinnamon that will teach you its benefits and also how to use it effectively in your daily life. As you will see once you reach the end, cinnamon is a humble spice that can be incorporated into your daily consumption without disrupting normalcy.

Cinnamon is nature at its most benevolent, and its benefits will leave you wondering what other secrets Mother Nature holds!

Getting Started

Chapter # 1: Intro

Before going into the details of the various health benefits of cinnamon, it is a good idea to provide a summary introduction to this spice for those who may be unaware of what it is.

Cinnamon is a spice, derived from the bark of several trees belonging to the Cinnamomum genus that is well-known among kitchens and chefs around the world. Almost everyone has tasted cinnamon rolls, cinnamon toast or at the very least cinnamon flavored gum.

The species Cinnamomum verum is considered to be the original 'true cinnamon' whereas many other types of cinnamon exist which are derived from other species of the genus. These are called 'cassia' to separate them from true cinnamon.

Many names have been given to cinnamon over the ages and by different cultures: the Greeks knew it as *kinnámōmon*, the Sri Lankans called it *kurundu*, to the Tamil it was *karuva*, and among the Javanese and Sumatrans it was referred to as *kayu manis* which is the local phrase used to describe sweet-tasting bark.

As stated previously, there are numerous types of cinnamon available in the market and even among each species; there can be several different types on the basis of the flavor of the bark of the tree from which it is extracted.

The unique flavor of cinnamon is due to an aromatic essential oil that makes up around one percent (but no more) of its composition. It gives the cinnamon its characteristic odor and spicy, fragrant flavor. This oil can be extracted from the cinnamon bark and is yellow when seen separately. This essential oil consists about ninety percent of a chemical compound known as a 'cinnamaldehyde' to which it owes its signature flavor.

Cinnamon trade flourished in the ancient world and continues to do so up to this day. Today, Sri Lanka is the world's largest producer of true cinnamon.

As a matter of interest, cinnamon was extremely coveted among ancient civilizations where it was often presented to kings and monarchs as a gift and was even deemed fit by many cultures as an offering to the gods. The Hebrew Bible contains a mention of this spice in several of its passages.

Today, science has uncovered many of its benefits that justify the reverence placed by the ancient peoples on this humble spice.

Chapter # 2: How is cinnamon commonly used?

There are a number of reasons why cinnamon has become so popular around the world.

The most obvious one is its pungent taste and aroma that is used by chefs around the world to liven up the cuisine they serve. Its naturally pleasant and invigorating smell can boost the attractiveness of any dish.

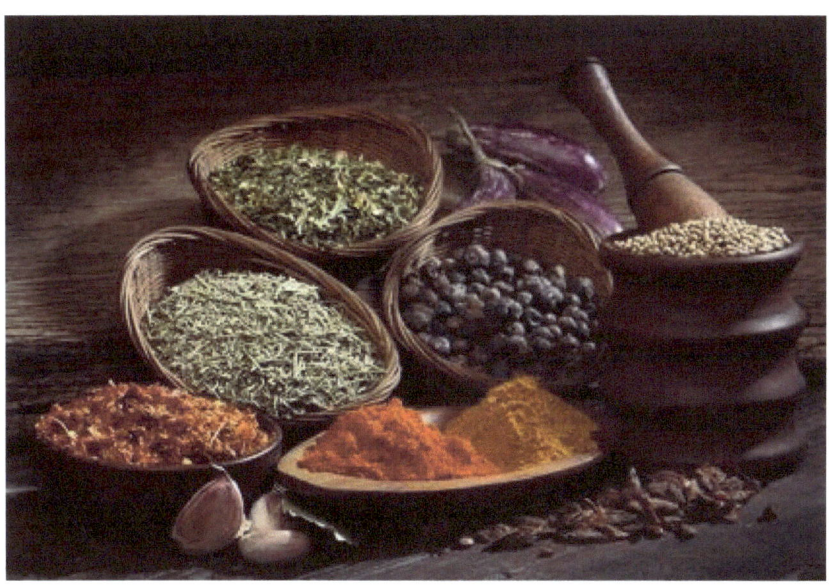

Besides this, cinnamon is used by herbalists and naturalist because of its powerful medicinal properties that range from fighting bacteria to combating cancer.

The direct health benefits notwithstanding, cinnamon has a number of properties that affect human health in a number of subtle ways. Its aroma can be inculcated in dry or simmering potpourri to liven up the fragrance of your home, ground cinnamon and essential oil of cinnamon can both be used as air fresheners and incense that can greatly curb your bad mood and stress.

As if that wasn't enough, cinnamon can be used as an insect repellent and its essential oil is particularly effective against mosquitoes.

Chapter # 3: Types of cinnamon

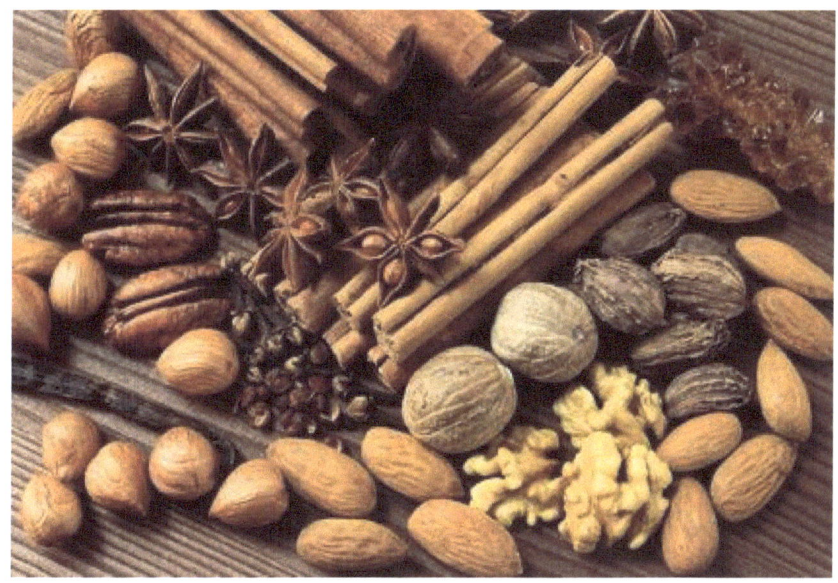

There is a diverse range of cinnamon that is cultivated and sold throughout the world. However, all types of cinnamon are derived from the bark of specie of the genus Cinnamomum. There is differentiation within each specie as well, based on factors such as the strength of its flavor. Cinnamon is loosely divided into two categories:

> **Cinnamomum verum:**

Also known as true cinnamon or Ceylon cinnamon (because of the fact that it is cultivated mostly in Sri Lanka, formerly Ceylon) is of superior quality to the other variety because of its subtler and more delicate flavor. Ceylon contains negligible traces of coumarin – a compound that is present in all cinnamon and is harmful for the lever. Its bark is thin; it is a lighter shade of brown and has a light and crumbly texture. This variety of the spice may be known as true cinnamon but it isn't the one that is consumed by the majority of the world's population. The reason in most cases is simple: it is more expensive. There are several subdivisions of true cinnamon due to variations in the taste of its bark: *Pani Kurundu, Pat Kurundu or Mapat Kurundu, Naga Kurundu, Pani Miris Kurndu, Weli Kurundu, Sewala Kurundu, Kahata Kurundu, Pieris Kurundu* from Type 1 through Type 7 Sinhala respectively.

➢ **Cassia cinnamon:**

This is the collective name given to the species:

C. burmannii or Indonesian cinnamon is known as Padang cassia and is one of the cheapest cinnamon spices available in the US market. C. loureiroi or Saigon cinnamon is called Vietnamese cassia and has the greatest oil percentage of cinnamaldehyde among all the cinnamon species which accounts for its higher price than several other varieties. It is an integral part of Vietnamese cuisine. C. cassia or Chinese cinnamon is the original Chinese cassia against which the other non verum species of the spice are compared. It is of a reddish brown appearance and its bark is thicker and coarser than the other varieties and consequently is also harder to grind. Its flavor is harsher than Ceylon cinnamon which is why it is less expensive too. It is the most abundantly available cinnamon in the US.The problem with cassia cinnamon is more than just its decidedly less subtle flavor: it has a larger percentage content of the toxic compound coumarin, which is why it is regarded as more harmful for human consumption than true cinnamon. When buying cinnamon at a market, make it a preference to purchase true cinnamon since its flavor is more pleasant and it carries a lower risk of damaging your liver because of its lower coumarin content.

Chapter # 4: Making the most of cinnamon in daily life

This section covers some general tips that will help you use cinnamon to full effect in your routine life without abusing it. You will be able to maximize the beneficial effects of the spice by following the advice in this section and keep its harmful effects to a minimum.

1. **Buy fresh, keep fresh:** The most important factor in maximizing the potency of this spice is its freshness. It is available in the market as a powder or in the form of quills, and ought to be treated gently in order to ensure that it doesn't lose its flavor or aroma. When you buy cinnamon keep in mind that ground cinnamon stays free for a half a year whereas cinnamon sticks keep their freshness for a full year. Seal it in a glass jar and store it in a cool and dry place to keep it fresh for longer periods of time; used cans work equally well. The spice's shelf life can be improved by refrigerating its container.
   The easiest way to check for the freshness of cinnamon is to smell it to see if it tastes sweet. If it has lost its characteristic aroma, then obviously, it has gone stale.

2. **Buy organically grown cinnamon:** You should go for cinnamon that has been grown in natural gardens to ensure that it hasn't been sprayed or irradiated. Irradiation can cause cinnamon to lose some of its Vitamin C or carotenoid content.

3. **Consume cinnamon sparingly in foods:** It is a good idea to include this spice in some of the foods you consume on a regular base. The quantity can range between one and six grams per day and is enough for you to benefit from the positive properties of cinnamon. You can include cinnamon in baked foods such as cakes, pastries or bread, or sprinkle it on your soups and stews. Remember that this spice combines with hot food much better than cold ones, and although its benefits are same for both, consuming foods containing unmixed cinnamon can be slightly difficult for some.

4. **Combine cinnamon in a warm drink:** One or two teaspoons of ground cinnamon in your tea, coffee or soup can be an excellent way to incorporate this spice into your diet and will greatly help in alleviating the symptoms of cold and flu. An added bonus is the uniquely pleasant flavor it lends to the drinks.

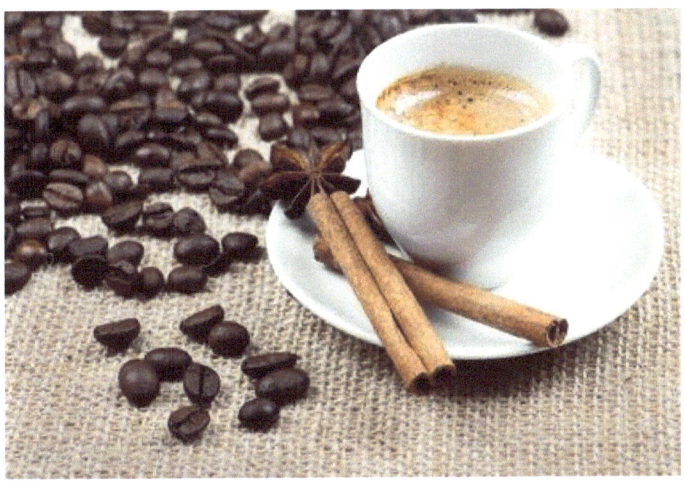

5. **Cinnamon after meals:** Cinnamon consumed after meals can aid people with weak digestive systems by stimulating their gastric juices. So if you suffer from heart burn or indigestion try a cup of cinnamon tea after dinner.

6. **Cinnamon can help when you're on a diet:** A cinnamon seasoning on foods with high carbohydrate content can lower their impact on your blood sugar levels. This has been proven by extensive research, so if you're on a diet and want to consume the occasional high crab treat, try it with a dash of cinnamon added to it. However, diabetics will do well to remember that cinnamon is not a substitute for insulin and should not be used as such. In fact, it is best to consult your doctor about the impact cinnamon may have on your blood sugar levels before you start to consume it.

7. **Chew cinnamon flavored gum:** Chewing cinnamon flavored gum, or even a simple whiff of cinnamon, can have a positive effect on the brains cognitive process. This is a good idea if you're a student or you have a job that requires constant presence of mind. You may even keep a bowl of ground cinnamon at your office as a natural air freshener that doubles as a mind booster! Remember that commercial cinnamon flavored air fresheners won't get the job done since they will most probably be artificial.

8. **Use cinnamon in soups and drinks instead of baked goods:** Cinnamon has the ability reduce the risk of heart disease and can also improve the working of the colon. However, if you keep consuming cinnamon cakes and cookies in the hope that the cinnamon will negate the effects of the carbs completely, you'll be getting nowhere. For the specific purpose of combating heart disease, it is a good idea to consume cinnamon in drinks and soups, and cut down on the carbs!

9. **Cinnamon is an anticoagulant:** The active oil cinnamaldehyde present in cinnamon can decrease the clumping of blood platelets in your stream. This can be harmful for those with blood disorders since higher than recommended levels of cinnamon can lead to uncontrolled bleeding among some patients. Also, if you have a surgery coming up in the near future, stay away from foods containing cinnamon as the reduced platelet levels it causes can prolong the aftermath of the surgery.

10. **Intake cinnamon through the air you breathe:** Apart from consuming cinnamon in drinks, you can use it as an extremely effective room freshener. Potpourris can be incorporated with cinnamon to produce an extremely pleasant aroma or it can be used simply as a ground powder.

With so many ways to make cinnamon a part of your life there is hardly any reason why you shouldn't do so- especially when it is so unobtrusive and beneficent.

Chapter # 5: Maximum daily dosage

The compound coumarin has been regarded as toxic by the European Food Safety Authority because of its adverse effects on the liver and kidneys in higher concentrations. Since it is a considerable constituent of cinnamon, a maximum recommended Tolerable Daily Intake of one tenth of milligram has been confirmed. The EU has enforced limits on the amount of coumarin that can be present in food and the levels of coumarin stated in these limits have been so low as to have a noticeable effect on the quantity of cinnamon present in pastries!

Benefits of cinnamon to the brain

Chapter # 6: Boosts brain activity

Cinnamon could have an enhancing effect on the brain according to a research conducted by the Wheeling Jesuit University in the US. The research team headed by Dr P. Zoladz, has reported that cinnamon when consumed as a flavoring or as when inhaled boosted the participants' brain functions related to attention, virtual recognition, working memory and visual motor reaction rate.

The research was conducted in a two pronged manner. Participants' brain functions were tested by means of a computer program after they had consumed various flavors of chewing gums. Among the flavors was cinnamon. In the second phase, they were tested after they had inhaled four odors, again, one of which happened to be cinnamon.

The results showed a clear relationship between the efficiency with which the participants carried out the tasks and the enhancing effect of the various odors and flavors. In particular, the results pointed out that cinnamon had the strongest bolstering effect on the efficiency with which the tasks were carried out, in terms of both flavor and aroma.

The preliminary implications of these findings are that the food industry has a new type of functional food that could be used to enhance memory of those who consume it. This means that when you're eating a cinnamon flavored chewing gum (that actually contains real cinnamon flavor) you'll be giving your brain a boost.

These findings prove that you do not have to get a particular brain enhancing drug prescribed to you if you feel that your brain's memory function is declining. By simply taking a whiff of cinnamon before a test, you will be able to do it better.

Chapter # 7: Protects against Alzheimer's disease

Alzheimer's disease is a name that runs synonymous with progressive dementia – in fact; it is the most common form of the later. Decades of research into this mental disorder have led to the development of no cure for this disease. It is the bane of the elderly and results in the complete breakdown of their day to day life.

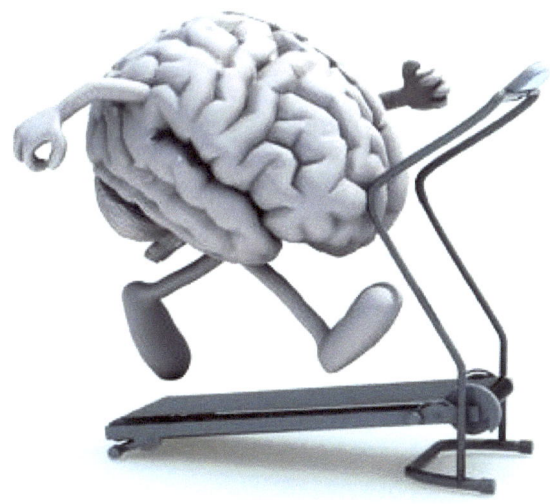

A new research however has infused hope within medical circles that cinnamon, the trivial spice used in cooking throughout the world, can delay the onset of or mitigate the effects of Alzheimer's. The secret lies in two compounds found in cinnamon's essential oil namely cinnamaldehyde and epicatechin that hold promise of being adversaries to the disease.

The findings of a study by two scientists at University of California – Santa Barbara, namely Roshni George and Donal Graves, Ph.D., were put forth in the Journal of Alzheimer's Disease's online issue. These two scientists believe that they can prove that the compounds mentioned above can block the formation of the filament like tangles that are present in brain cells characteristic of the disease.

Alzheimer's is also associated with the clumping together of a protein called tau. When this protein fails to bind properly, which is the case with Alzheimer's patients, these clumps are formed and their knots and tangles get progressively worse as the disease sets in. However, cinnamaldehyde has proved itself effective in the prevention of these tau knots. In layman's terms, cinnamaldehyde works as a hat protects your face and head from oxidation: it binds itself to the cysteine residues of the tau protein, preventing its oxidation. Oxidation of the residues modifies their structure which contributes to the development of Alzheimer's.

The great thing is that cinnamaldehyde, while preventing the progression of Alzheimer's by protecting the tau protein, has no effect of its own on the protein. It can remove itself from the protein ensuring that there is no alteration in the protein's working.

The other compound, epicatechin, is a known powerful antioxidant which is in fact triggered by oxidation meaning that it can shield the cysteine residues of the tau protein in a manner similar to the action of the compound cinnamaldehyde. Furthermore, it takes care of the byproducts resulting from the oxidation of cell membranes which can also harm the cysteines.

Studies have indicated a strong link between diabetes and the occurrence of Alzheimer's disease. Again this is attributed to the fact that heightened blood glucose levels that are found in diabetics can lead to excessive formation of oxidants that cause oxidative stress in the brain. It is already well established that cinnamon is helpful in managing blood glucose levels in diabetics, so this too indicates an indirect aid in dealing with Alzheimer's.

The researcher have advised readers not to take this as a signal to start consuming more cinnamon than is the daily recommended dose since its excess can harm the liver and kidneys.

Benefits of cinnamon to the body

Chapter # 8: Regulates blood sugar

According to an ongoing research, cinnamon has shown itself as potent natural agent in the fight against diabetes.

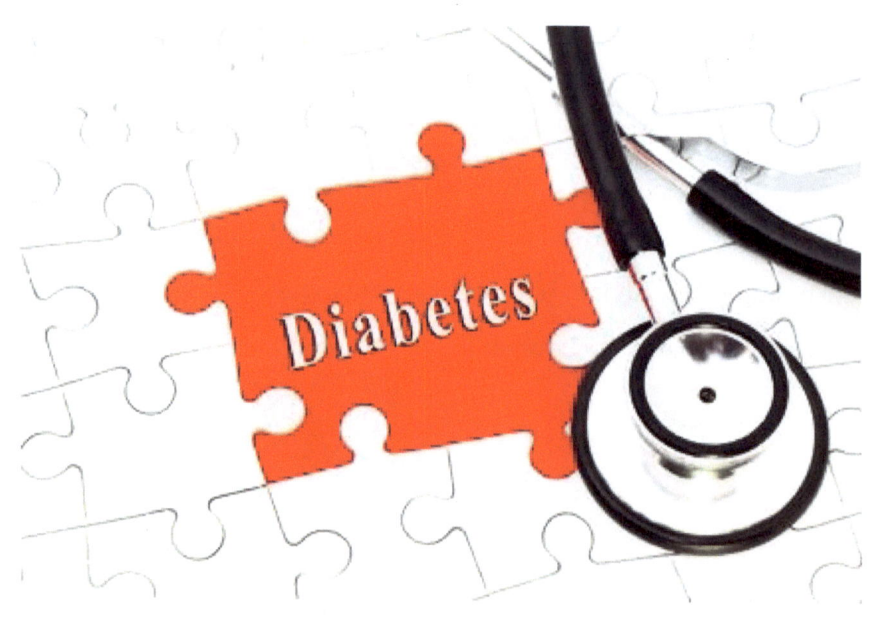

The most significant of cinnamon's effects on those with diabetes is the apparent reduction in blood sugar levels it triggers, even a dosage as small as one half tbsp. Cinnamon has shown considerable results in this department. This is good news for diabetics who can include a minimal amount of cinnamon in their regular diet to benefit from this property of cinnamon.

Here are some of the ways by which cinnamon controls your blood sugar:

1. It raises your glucose metabolism rate by twenty times which obviously improves the regulation of your blood sugar.
2. It has a bioactive compound that gives it effects similar to that of the hormone insulin which is crucial in maintaining your blood sugar levels.
3. It reduces the rate at which your stomach empties and thus controls rapid rises in sugar levels after meals.
4. It also enhances the sensitiveness of insulin and a bioflavinoid known as proanthocyanidin, which may be responsible for altering the insulin signaling action in fat cells.

Chapter # 9: Aids in weight loss

Due to the regulatory effect it has on blood sugar levels and the way it imitates and stimulates insulin levels in the body, cinnamon is well known for the aid it lends to those looking to lose some weight. Indeed, it has been consumed as a natural weight loss agent for a long time. Because cinnamon enhances the rate at which glucose is metabolized, it indirectly reduces the amount of fat present in the body since high sugar levels can be the cause of increased fat content in the body.

That's not all, cinnamon changes the very manner in which the metabolism of sugar occurs in your body and stops it from turning into fat.

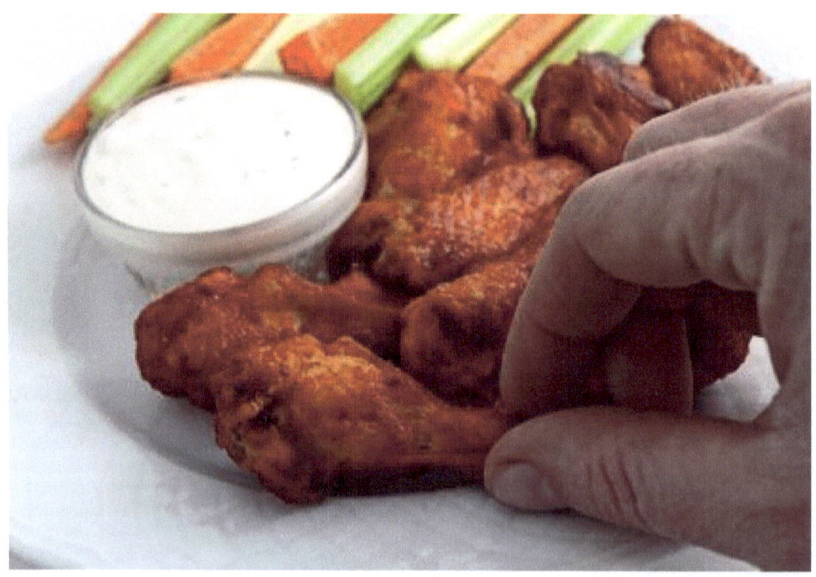

As was previously mentioned, it slows down the rate at which food passes out of your stomach meaning that it helps keep you from getting hungry too quickly. Thus, it is a great additive in the diets of those who want to lose weight since it puts a stop to their constant cravings for food. It also aids the body in the processing of carbs which also helps in weight loss.

Studies indicate that fat present in the abdominal region of our bodies is more susceptive to the effects of cinnamon than that present in other regions.

Chapter # 10: Helps fight cancer

Researchers at the United States Department of Agriculture in Maryland have published a study that gives strong evidence of cinnamon's ability to fight cancer growth. The scientists used powdered cinnamon made into a water soluble extract for their research.

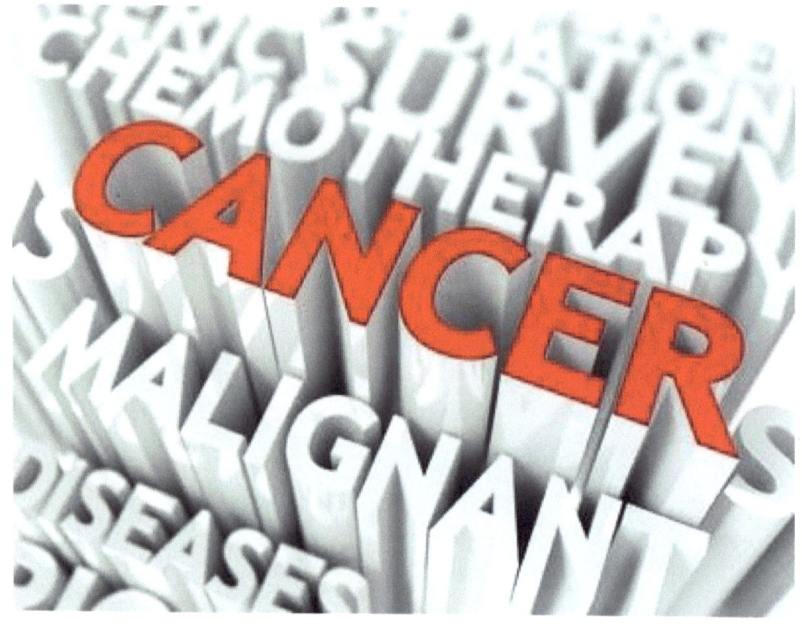

The anti-cancer effects of cinnamon are attributed to some of its compounds that mimic the hormone insulin and help control type two diabetes. They are called procyanidins. Additionally, a polymeric compound called methylhydroxychalcone or simply MHCP also has insulin like properties. These compounds are collectively a part of *polymeric polyphenols* i.e. they consist of a chain of molecules, each of which holds more than one *phenol*. These plant polyphenols have antioxidant properties that, for the larger part, grant them the ability to protect against different types of cancer. However, some scientists are of the opinion that these compounds have other properties as well that can account completely for their anti-cancer abilities. These may be the limiting or stimulating of enzymes that take part in the growth of cells in the human body.

The researchers applied the cinnamon extract to three types of cancerous human cells: two of which represented leukemia and one to account for lymphoma. These two diseases are responsible for the harmful growth of blood cells and lymph cells respectively.

The results were collected after period of twenty four hours and were positively astounding. The water-soluble cinnamon extract decreased the rate of cancerous cell growth by a drastic amount and this effect was proportional to the dose of cinnamon extract administered. At the maximum dose, the cell count showed that the cancerous cells in the cinnamon administered culture were 50% less than control cancer cell culture. This means that the seemingly insignificant spice practically halted the proliferation of cancer cells!

Apparently, cinnamon halts the cell division by limiting the working of some certain phosphate enzymes that are vital in cell reproduction.

This research has also indicated a relationship between diabetes and cancer since the same compounds that help in the fight against diabetes also facilitate in the struggle against cancer. This has prompted several researches to focus on a potential link between excessive production of insulin and the onset of cancer.

Chapter # 11: Combats infertility

A small study conducted by a group of researchers at the Columbia University Medical Center in NYC has reported that cinnamon helps in alleviating the effects of a feminine health condition called polycystic ovary syndrome. The study showed that women who ingested small amounts of cinnamon on a daily basis over a span of six months reported twice as many menstrual cycles as those who did not.

By countering the menstrual irregularity caused by this condition, this inexpensive spice helps reduce infertility in women. Indeed, two of the women who were subjects in the research reported pregnancies during the research phase.

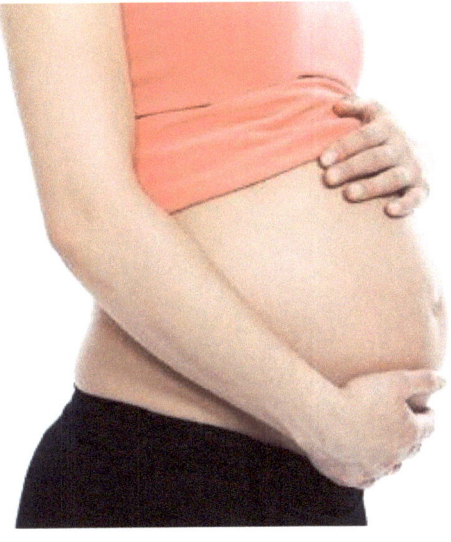

Polycystic ovary syndrome is believed to result from the body's insensitivity to the hormone insulin and since cinnamon is known to incorporate compounds that imitate the effects of insulin and sensitize it as well, there is a strong argument in favor of its effects against polycystic ovary syndrome.

The research, though giving a strong indication of a relationship between the spice and betterment of polycystic ovary syndrome, was unable to pinpoint the exact constituent of cinnamon that affects the condition.

Chapter # 12: Reduces arthritic pain

Arthritis is a painful condition of the joints of the knees that can put many a healthy person to bed. A research conducted at the Copenhagen University has shown that a mixture of one tbsp. honey and half tbsp. cinnamon powder taken daily before breakfast can work wonders in alleviating the pain of those suffering from chronic arthritis. One week into the research, a third of the patients being treated were completely relieved of their pain and one month from the start of the trial, nearly all the patients whose movement had been impaired by the sever arthritic pain were once again able to walk.

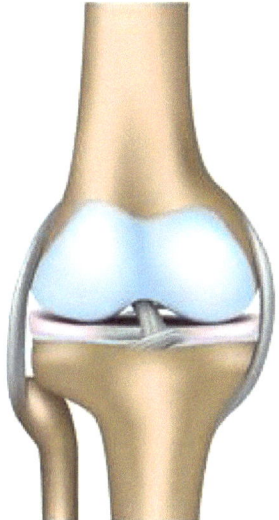
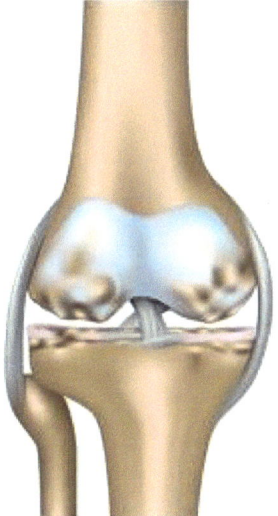

Healthy knee joint   Osteoarthritis

For best results, arthritis patients are recommended to drink a cup of hot water mixed with two tbsp. of honey and one tbsp. of cinnamon powder daily, day and night. However, it should be remembered that cinnamon in large quantities can be toxic so it is best to use Ceylon cinnamon that contains lesser toxic content. Moreover, ensuring that the honey is completely natural is also a good idea. Needless to say, honey contains a lot of natural sugar so it shouldn't be taken in excess. Just follow the dosage mentioned above and you will be fine!

Chapter # 13: Has inherent anti-infectious properties

Ancient medicine has used a mixture of honey and cinnamon in the treatment of sore throat and infections. Today, science has proven that cinnamon has the ability to fight infections caused by a multitude of bacteria, fungi and viruses.

The key to the infection warding properties of cinnamon lies in its bark whose biological function is to protect the plant from protection.

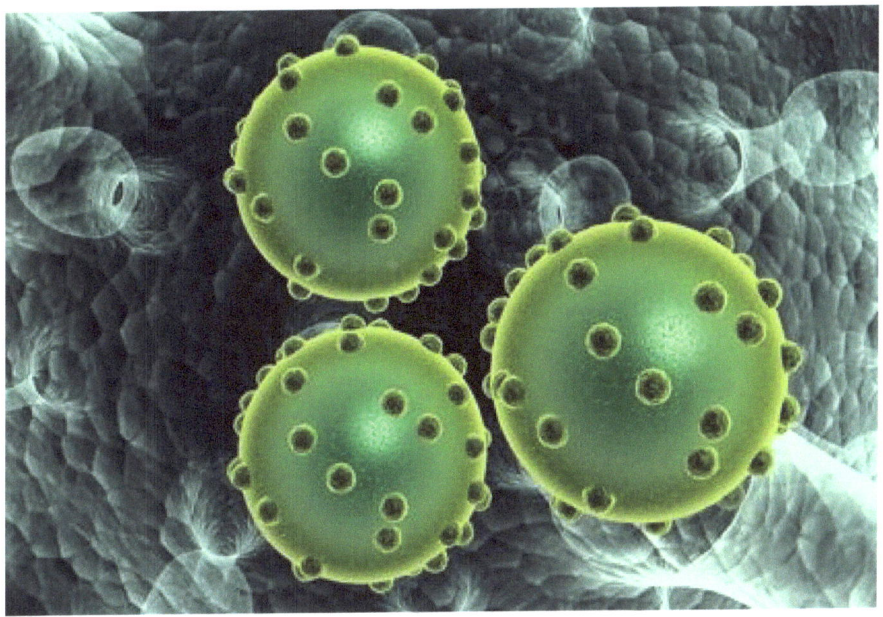

Here is a list of pathogens that cinnamon can shield the body from:

- Aspergillus niger

- Campylobacter Infections

- Candida Infection

- Coronaviridae (SARS-associated) Infections

- Escherichia coli Infections

- H1N1 Infection

- Head Lice

- HIV Infections

- Insect Bites: Repellent

- Klebsiella Infections

- Legionnaires' disease

- MRSA

- Pseudomonas aeruginosa

- Staphylococcal Infections

Cinnamon bark is composed of cinnamaldehyde which is known to be highly anti-viral in nature in addition to working against inflammation, soothing the nerves and widening the blood vessels. In large amounts it can be harmful so it shouldn't be consumed more than the maximum daily dosage. Additionally, cinnamon bark is, for the large part, composed of phenols, in particular eugenol, is a well reputed disinfectant, anesthetic and germ killer. Again, it should be taken sparingly since an excess can cause irritation in the skin and mucous membranes.

Chapter # 14: Helps against acne

The anti-bacterial, anti-inflammatory and antioxidant properties of cinnamon bark and oil can be effective against acne.

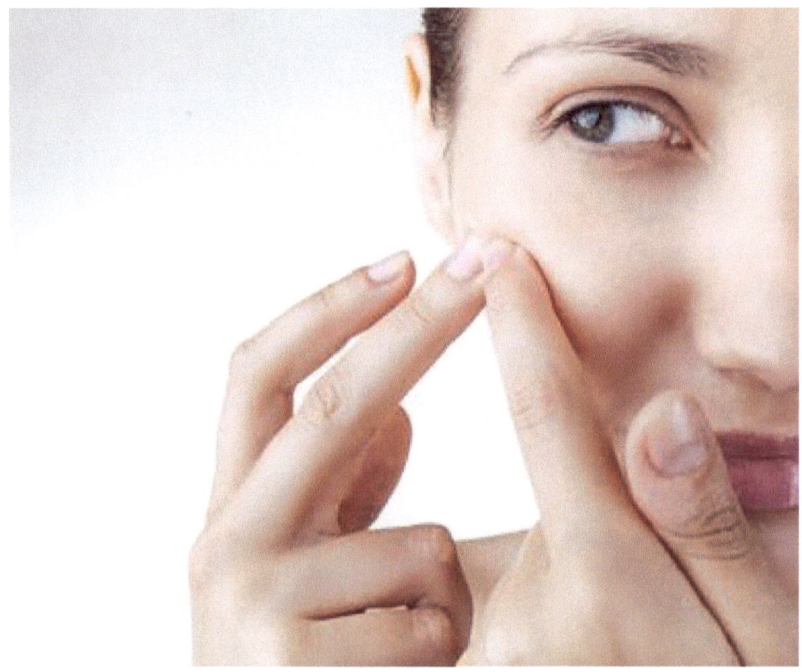

Cinnamon's anti-bacterial effect has been demonstrated by several researches conducted by reputed institutes and has been published in medical journals many times. The spice's anti-bacterial properties hold against the acne-causing microorganisms such as P. acnes and S. epidermis. Cinnamon oil can exterminate these bacteria present in the skin and thus prevent the pores from becoming clogged leading to a reduction in inflammation of the skin and sebum production caused by the bacteria.

A study conducted in 2002 has revealed that cinnamon has the ability to reduce the inflammation of the skin even more directly than by the procedure described above – it limits the formation of nitric oxide by inhibiting the enzyme nitric oxide synthase which speeds up the inflammation causing compound's production. This reduction in nitric oxide can result in decreased pimples, whiteheads and blackheads as well as acne lesions.

Cinnamon's antioxidant properties further shield the skin from the effects of toxins present in the environment and substances created as a result of the bacteria that get stuck in the pores of our skin. These substances are free radicals that damage follicles and skin proteins, but cinnamon can be used to remove them.

This isn't all; cinnamon powder has a microdermabrasion property which means it can remove the uppermost layer of dirt that gets accumulated as a result of the collective action of sebum, microorganisms and expired skin cells. This natural exfoliation is the courtesy of the extremely fine fiber characteristic of cinnamon powder.

Conclusion

By now, you will have been surprised at least once by the remarkable properties of this seemingly innocuous spice. What you considered as a pleasant flavor and aroma will be starting to seem like a miracle to you in its own right and you will most certainly be viewing it with a newfound reverence.

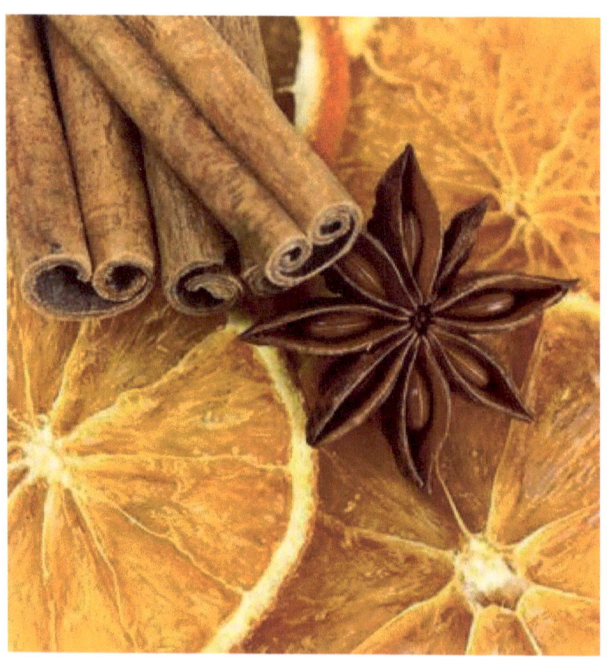

With powerful effects such as improving brain function, fighting diabetes and stopping the growth of cancerous cells, it is clear that cinnamon is a spice whose value isn't limited to the kitchen!

The integral role it plays in cuisine around the world only makes it easier to include this healthy spice into one's daily diet and take advantage of the numerous health benefits it has to offer.

However, the old saying, 'Excess of anything is bad', applies to cinnamon as well, so it should be taken in moderation, according to the daily dose recommended by international health authorities. When suffering from a specific medical condition, it will be a good idea to consult your physician before trying to make it a part of your diet.

Have fun trying out all the ways you can make cinnamon a part of your life!

Photo credits

1. http://us.fotolia.com/id/51347319

2. http://us.fotolia.com/id/47170066

3. http://us.fotolia.com/id/36637153

4. http://us.fotolia.com/id/58823942

5. http://www.fotolia.com/id/45156048

6. http://www.fotolia.com/id/39611032

7. http://www.fotolia.com/id/11347590

8. http://us.fotolia.com/id/49549245

9. http://www.fotolia.com/id/51669992

10. http://us.fotolia.com/id/38798477

11. http://us.fotolia.com/id/59321254

12. http://us.fotolia.com/id/54507728

13. http://us.fotolia.com/id/56287465

Author Bio

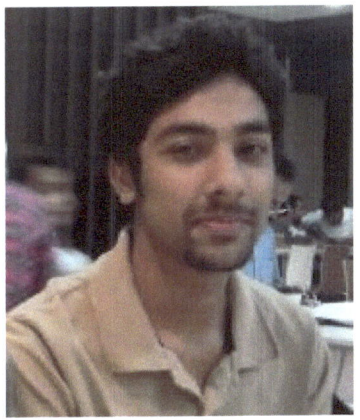

Muhammad Usman is a distinguished medical graduate of Allama iqbal medical college (AIMC). He is a professional writer who has been in the field for more than 4 years. During this time he has produced 10,000+ articles, blogs and eBooks on various niches related to diseases, health, fitness, nutrition and well being. He is a regular contributor to several journals related to medicine and surgery. He is the editor of several journals and newspapers.

Check out some of the other JD-Biz Publishing books

Gardening Series on Amazon

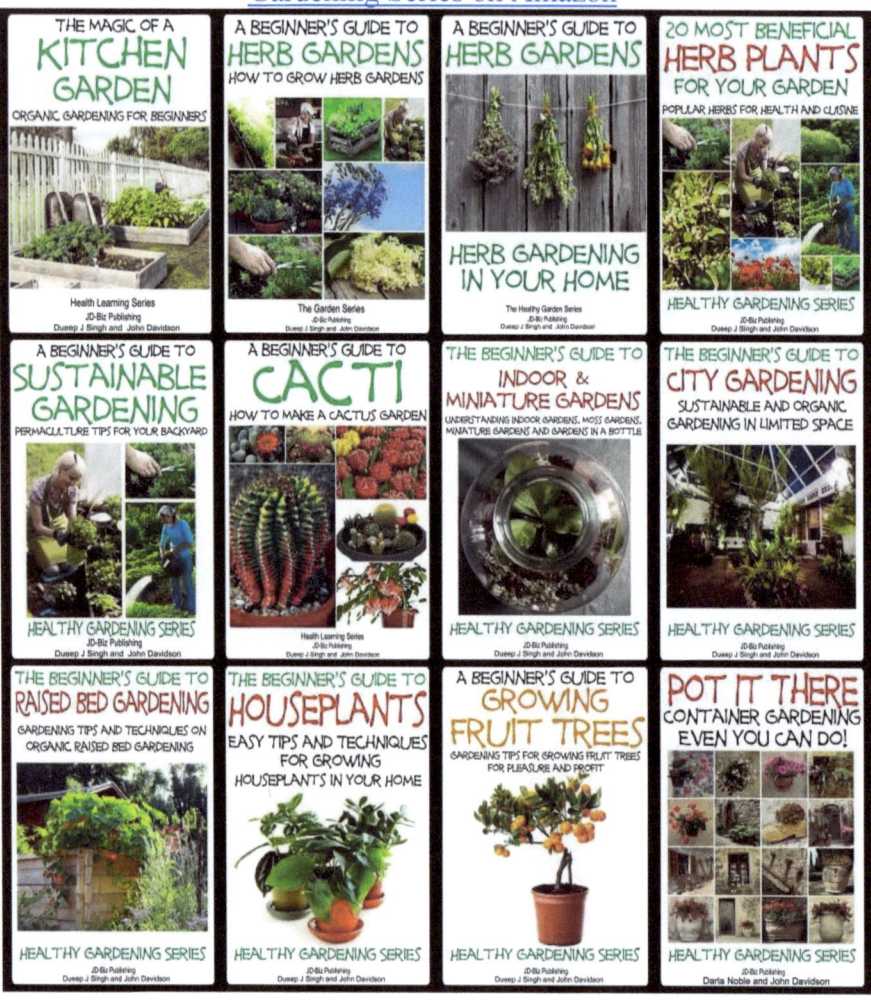

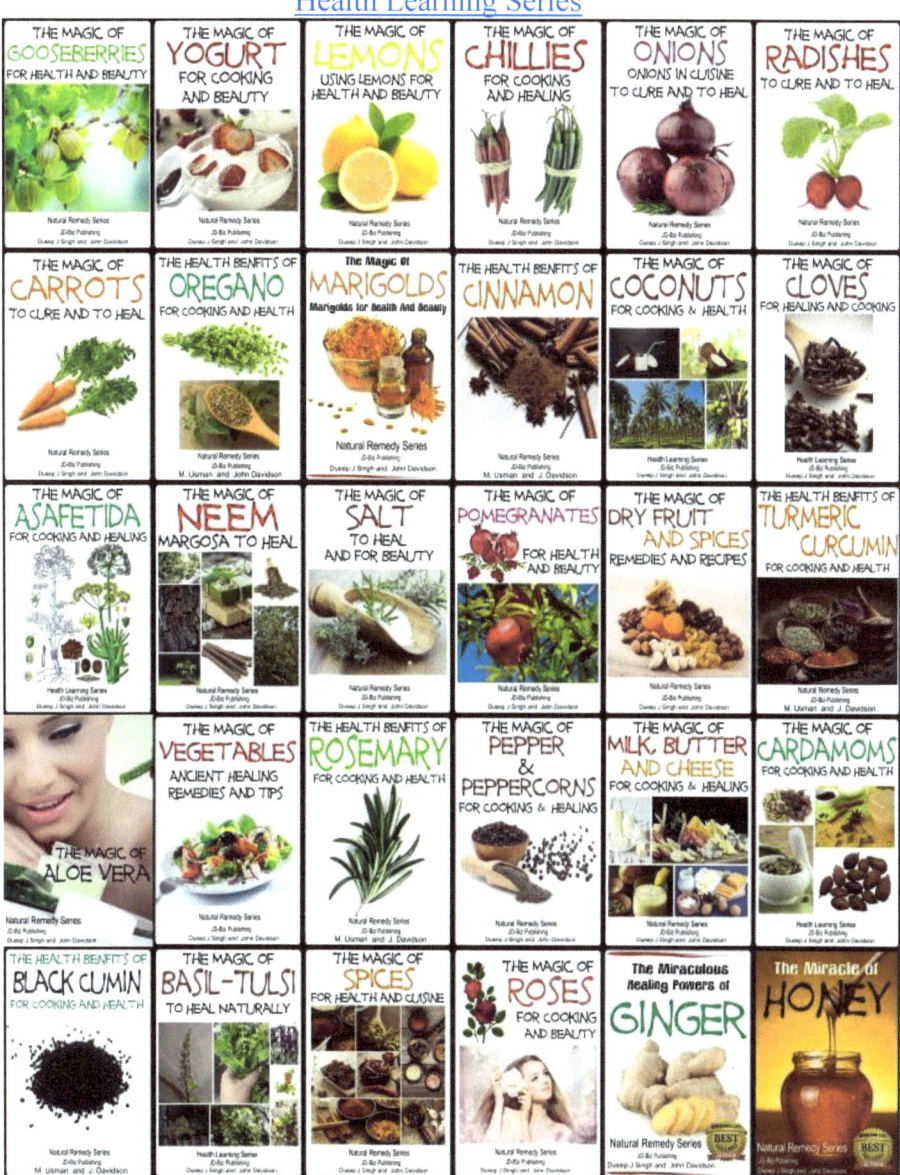

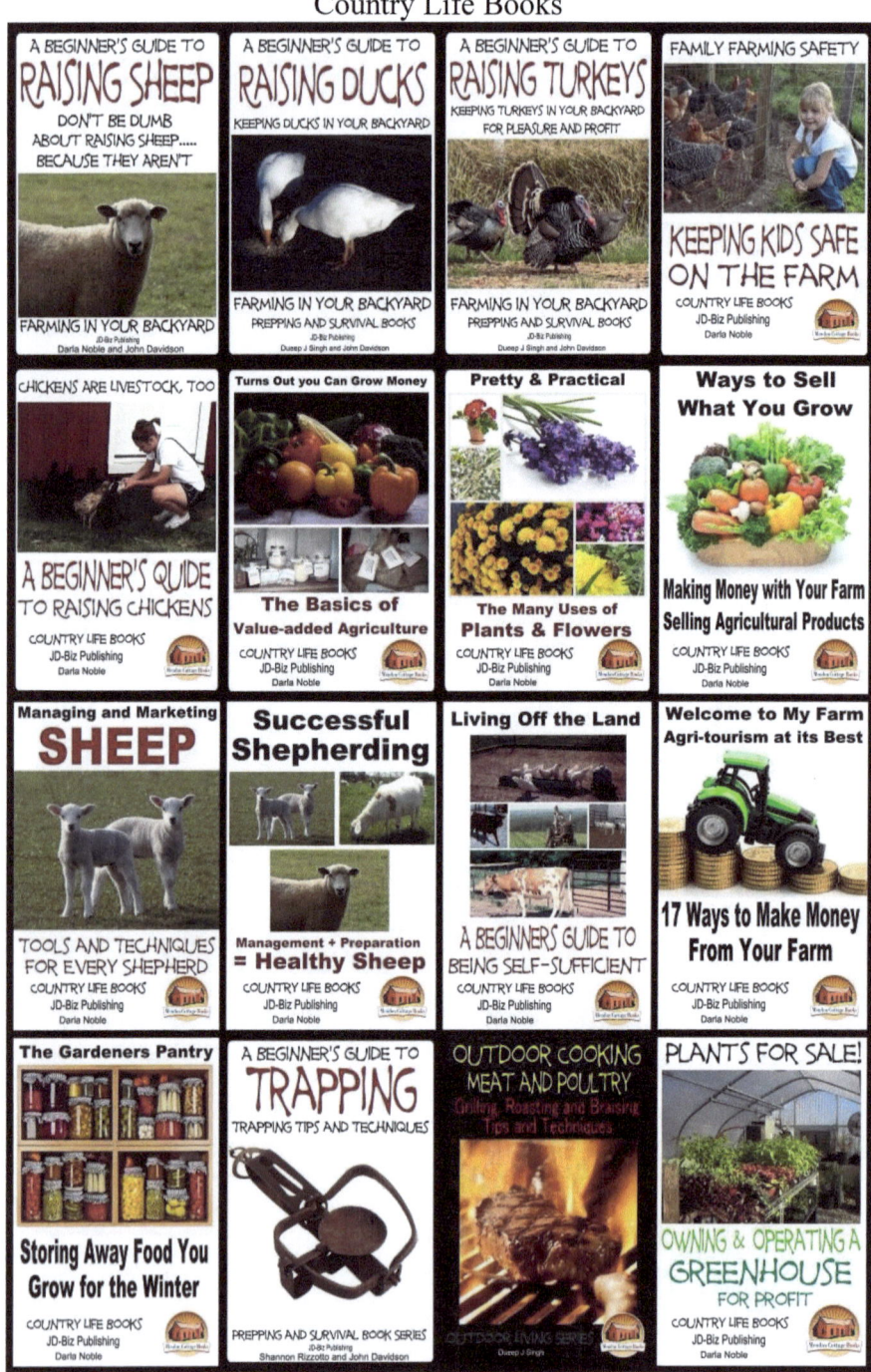

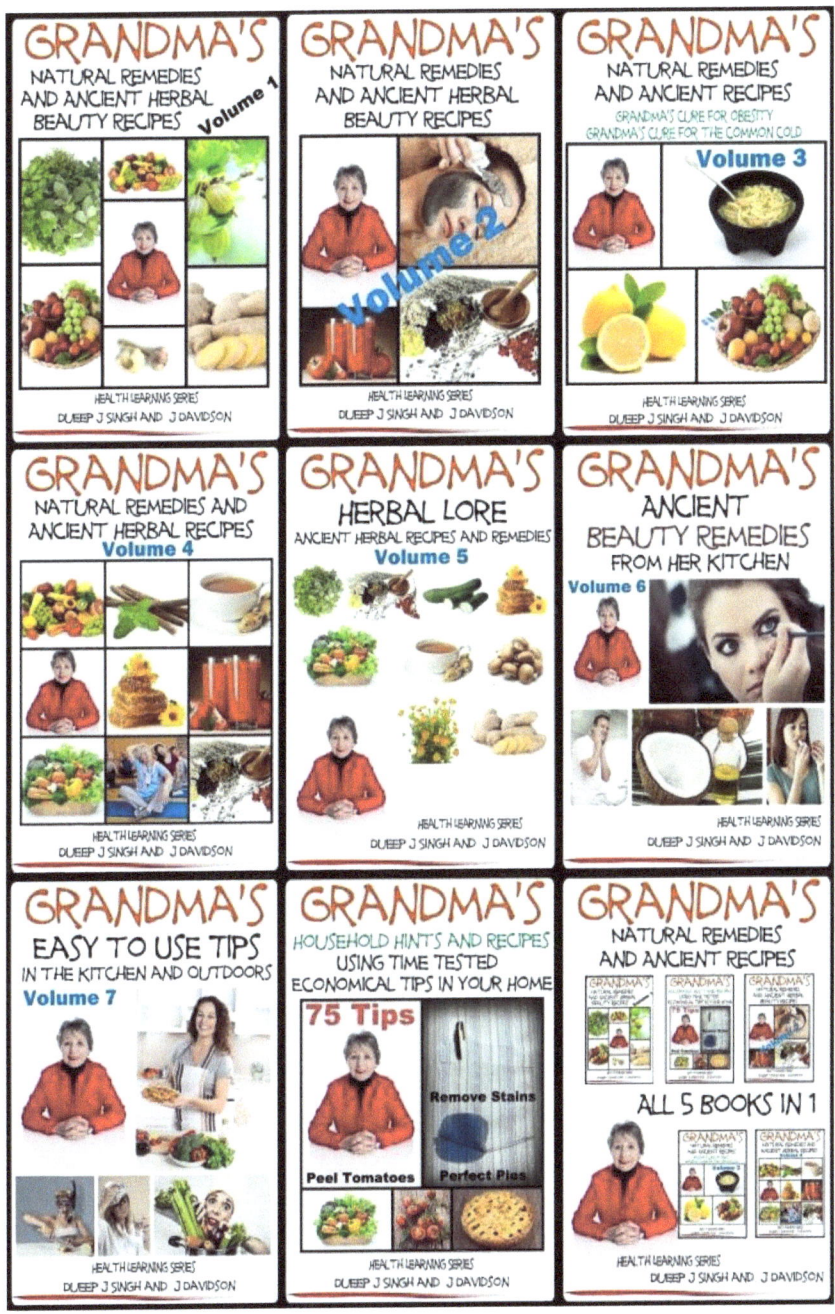

Health Learning Series

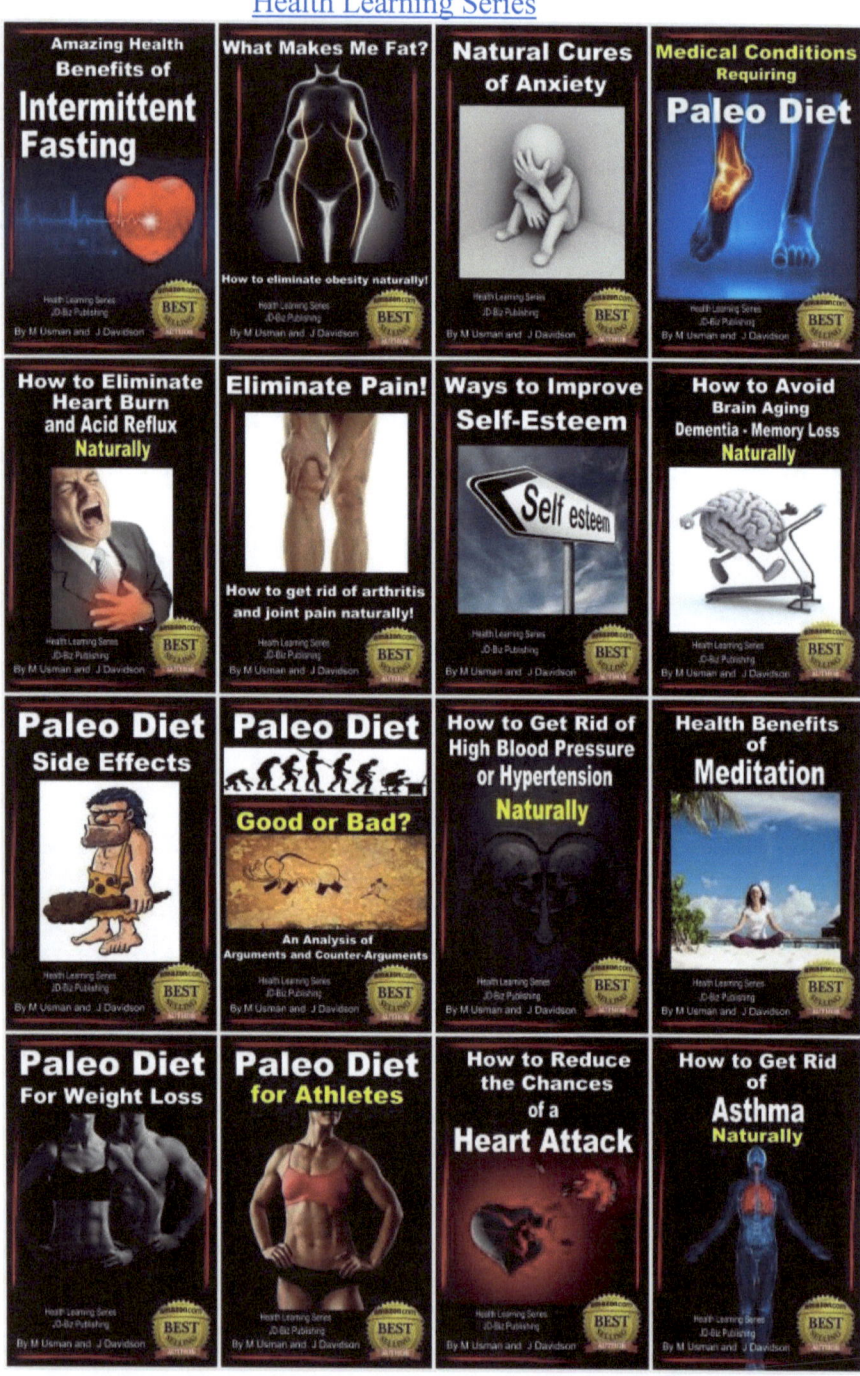

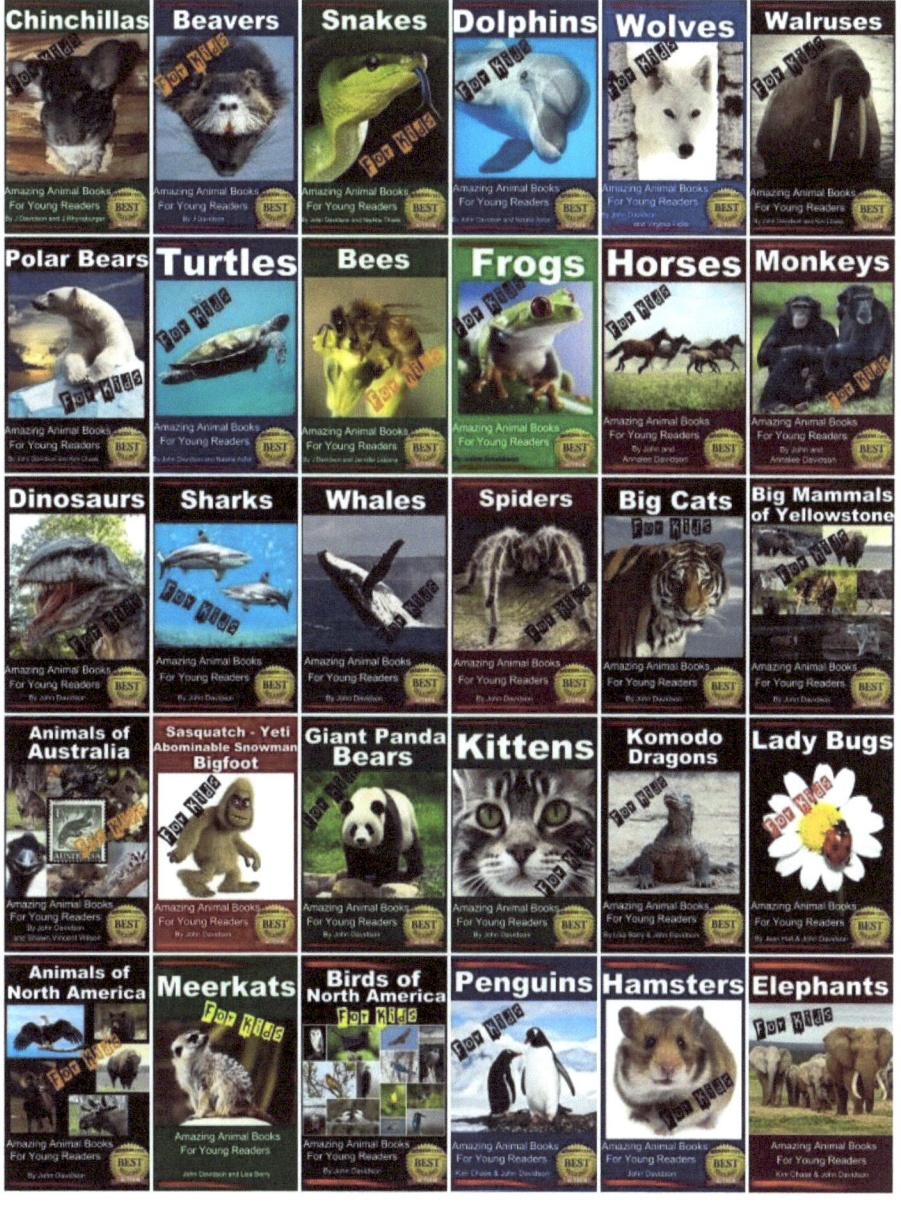

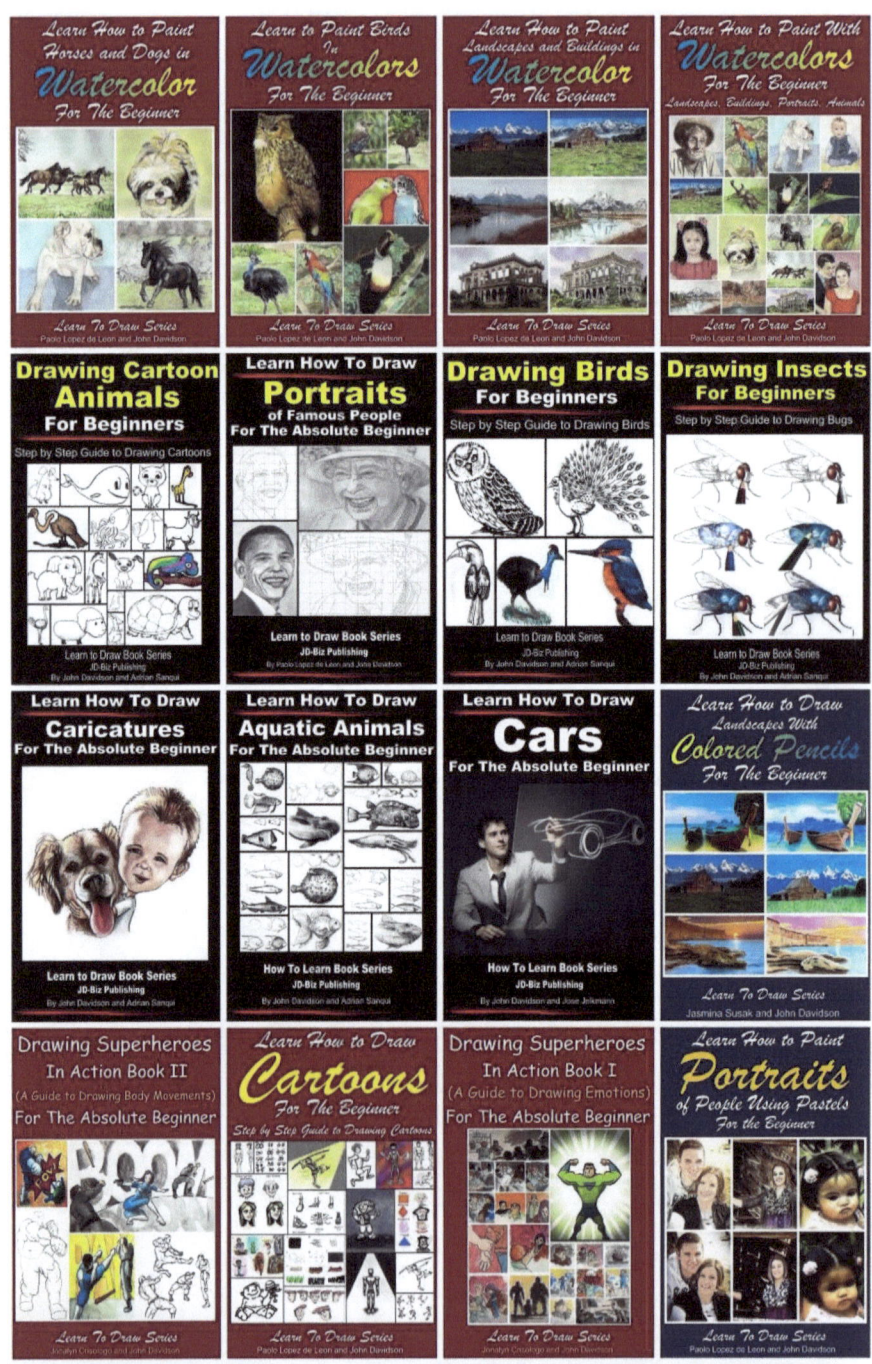

How to Build and Plan Books

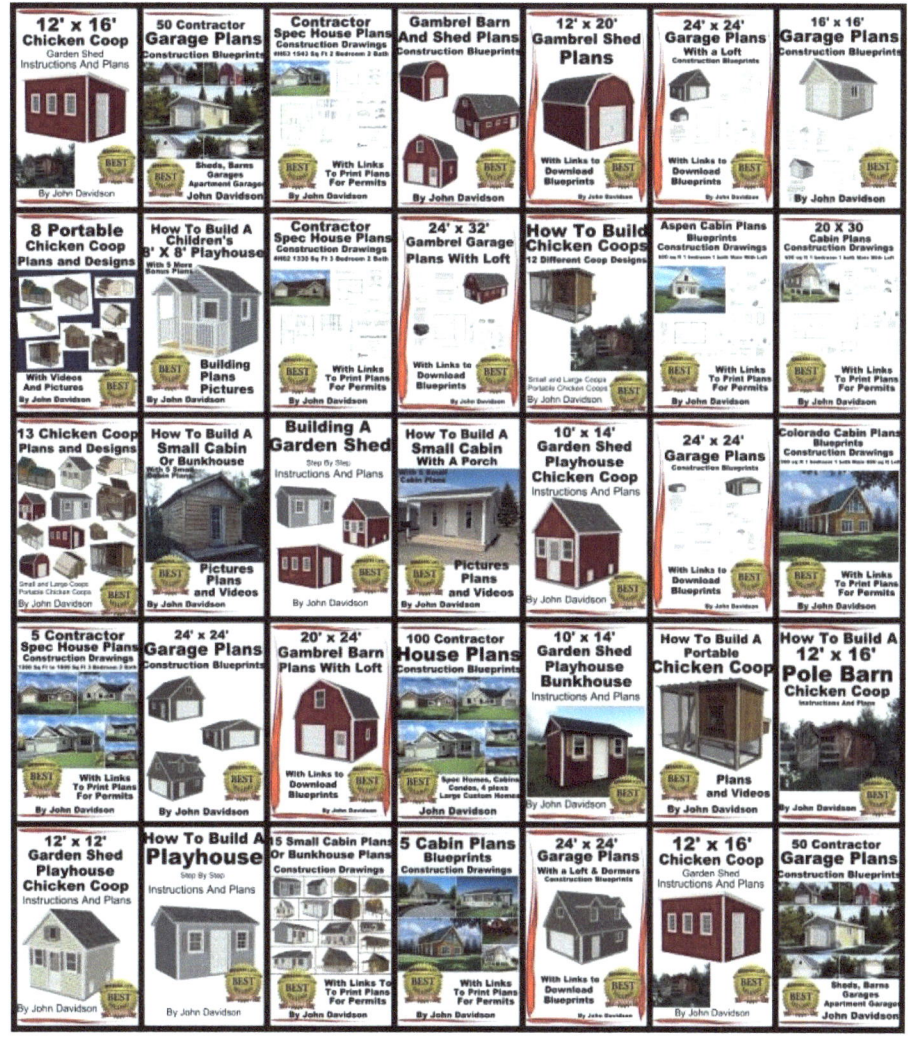

Entrepreneur Book Series

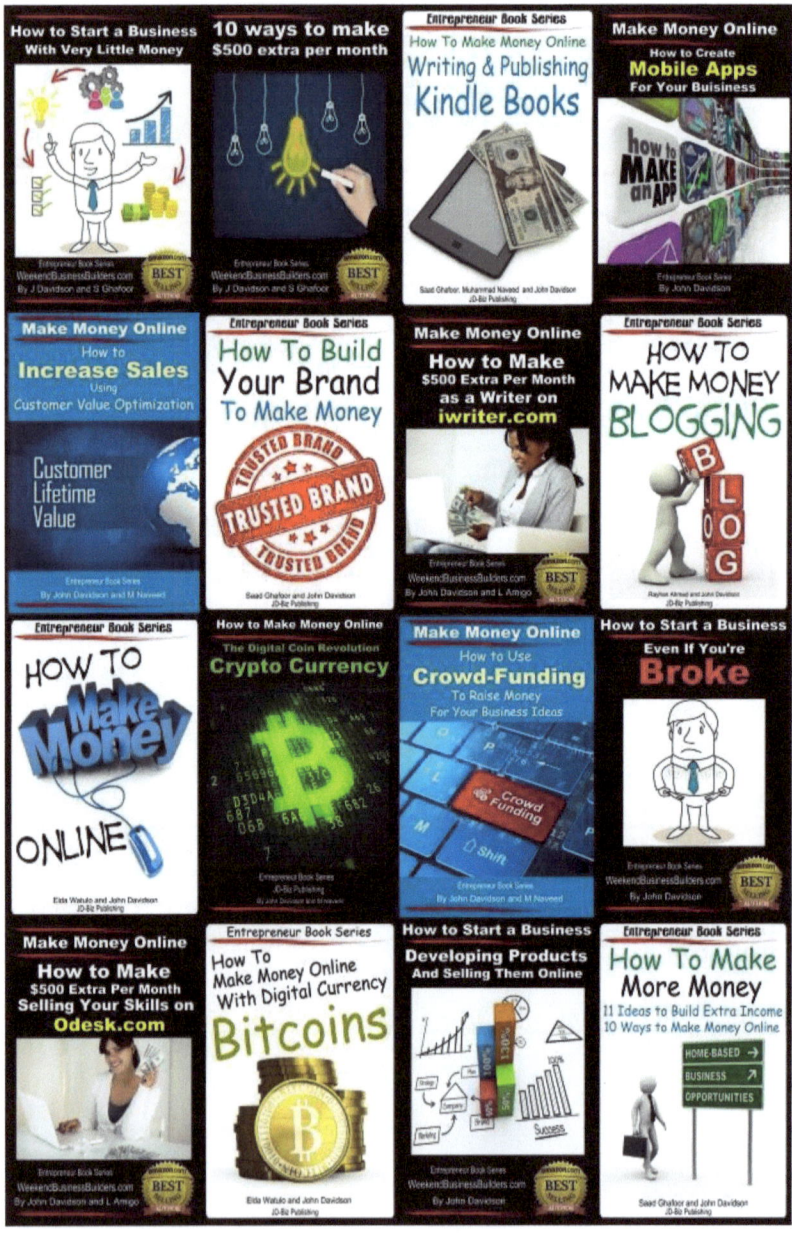

Our books are available at

1. Amazon.com

2. Barnes and Noble

3. Itunes

4. Kobo

5. Smashwords

6. Google Play Books

Download Free Books!

http://MendonCottageBooks.com

Publisher

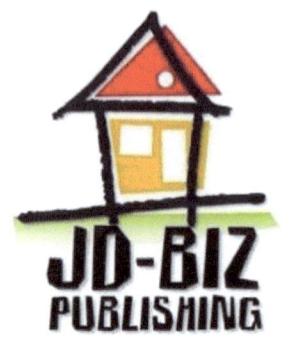

JD-Biz Corp

P O Box 374

Mendon, Utah 84325

http://www.jd-biz.com/

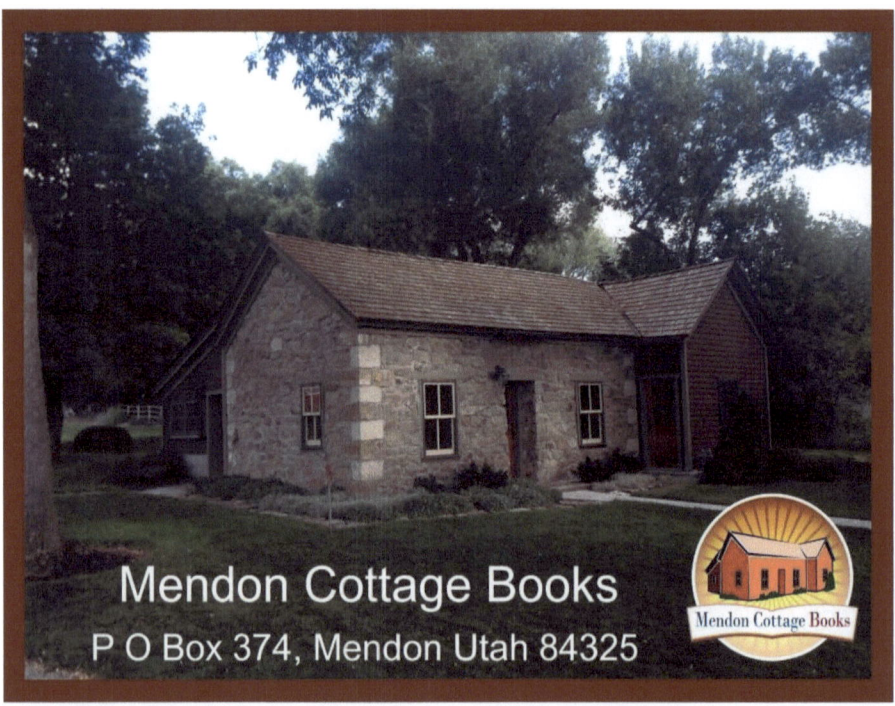

Mendon Cottage Books

P O Box 374, Mendon Utah 84325

www.ingramcontent.com/pod-product-compliance
Lightning Source LLC
Chambersburg PA
CBHW040313010626
45792CB00022B/288